Start the Revolution Within

START THE REVOLUTION WITHIN

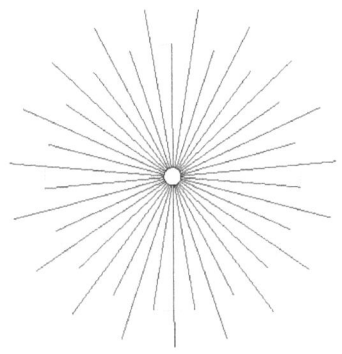

A Journey towards
Vibrant Health & Weight Loss

Transforming your
Body, Mind, Spirit & Emotions

Brian M Heater

Transformingourselves.com
www.transformingourselves.com
PO Box 3411 Ashland, OR 97520
541-261-7238

To my Mother and Father,
Jeanne & Marv Heater.

Their love and support is what brought me
to where I am today. I love you.

CONTENTS

Start the Revolution Within - Introduction

Section I –
The Connection Between
Body, Mind, Spirit & Emotions

Section I - Summary Worksheets

Section II –
The Natural Health & Weight Loss Program

Start the Revolution Within

Start the Revolution Within - Introduction

I want to share something with you. I feel great. I am blessed with how I feel. I am a new man. And I want you to feel this way also.

My life was not always great. At least I felt that way. In the past I have been negative, depressed, overweight and unhealthy. So this is a personal story. And it could possibly be your story as well. This is a story of transformation and hope. I am telling it to you because I want to help you. I feel a strong calling from the universe to write, to speak, anything I can do to get the word out that there is a better way of life which we all can have.

A year ago I was 315 lbs and unhealthy. I was overweight, around 70 lbs too heavy. I drank alcohol and ate food for comfort. I was negative and depressed. My attitude reflected my life as I fed into my unhealthy thinking. I constantly made excuses and blamed others for my problems. My finances were in ruin. I had just lost my house to foreclosure. This was one of the lowest points in my life.

I had not always been this low. I studied health, spirituality and had been a counselor for many years. I had many high points in my life and felt I had done some good work. Yet I felt there was something missing in my life. A lingering feeling that I was missing a key component of how to live a happy and fulfilling life.

This caused me to have intense lows. I also turned to external sources such as food, alcohol and drugs to comfort myself and find the answers. Little did I know how far I was from the truth. I knew in my heart and soul something had to change. I knew there was a better way to live. And I finally found the answers. So can you!

All of us go through the ups and downs of existence. This is part of our human experience. It is difficult to see, but your negative experiences are actually strengthening you to move on to the next level. Some people choose to move on, some of us don't. I was blessed in that I moved on to the next level. And if you need change, I want you to have the strength to move on also.

What I went through and continue to do was what many call an "awakening"….an opening up of my consciousness to all the present possibilities. A transformation of body, mind, spirit and emotions. I learned to let go of the past and focus on the present in all its pain and pleasure. I learned and continue to learn how to be happy to just live and experience life in the moment. I have learned gratitude and joy. This has changed my life.

I am a firm believer in the connection between body, mind, spirit and emotions. These four parts of us work together towards harmony. Ancient traditions and cultures understood these basic principles. The focus on the four elements (earth, air, water & fire) corresponded with the four parts of us. Living in harmony between these four elements was a basic part of their lives. We can incorporate those ancient beliefs with new ones of today. You need to have each part of yourself working in harmony. Sound body, mind, spirit and emotions are a key to your success and your happiness. You can't have one without the other. Some folks have a sound body and have worked hard towards that. This is wonderful. Yet if you focus on just the externals of ourselves, just that one part of yourself, you will not truly find permanent health and happiness.

We are at a crossroads as a society and as a world. And many of us feel this change. It is a great place to be right now and we should rejoice in the possibilities of growth and transformation. On the down side of this change is depression, anxiety and stress....a fast paced technological society. This is a major part of many people's lives. Many of us are overweight and unhealthy. Prescription drugs are given out like candy for all of our problems. We continue to eat unhealthy preservative laden junk foods. New fast food restaurants pop up everywhere. Illness is a major focus and topic.

What if I told you this could all go away? That your problems and stress are an illusion? That you are in control of your thoughts, feelings and beliefs? What if I told you that you could feel vibrant health and lose the permanent weight you desire? All these things can happen. They happened to me. Now they can happen to you.

I am here to tell you that life can change. That you are in control. You can be happy and feel a sense of joy in your life every day. I am not kidding you. I changed my life and feel great. I finally figured out the secret. I feel like a new man! I lost those 70 lbs I needed to get rid of and went on to lose another 13 lbs. I lost 83 lbs total! I became sober. I exercised daily. I meditated and focused myself on the power of the greater universe. I read and reread every book I could get my hands on that had to deal with health, attitude, science and spirituality. I went to counseling and learned techniques to help me let go of some past recordings in my mind. I set my goals, affirmed and visualized them every day. I believed in myself and in a higher power like no other time in my life. I visualized myself as being healthy and happy. I worked on each part of myself. I believe that it was the work on each part of me…body, mind, spirit and emotions that transformed my life. This is what this book and my program is all about.

So let's take this journey together. I'm going to discuss some important concepts with you. Things I have learned from countless others and through my own soul searching and my connection with the Divine, what scientists call the Zero Point Field, what some people call God, what others call the Universal Energy Field or Source Energy. Whatever your belief or terminology you use it does not really matter. What matters is for you to believe and to keep an open mind and become aware that there is energy everywhere. We, everything, is pure energy. We are connected to this and we can utilize this energy. We can transform our thoughts, feelings and actions. We can follow a basic universal principal called the "law of attraction". What you focus on manifests. You attract that which you think about. A positive thought is much stronger than you can imagine.

I want to teach you to take care of your body, mind, spirit and emotions. To find harmony. I'm going to give you some guidelines to live by. These guidelines are universal and cross all cultural and religious boundaries. These guidelines are the bridge which connect us all. They are not rules or steadfast dogma. They are general principles that can help you transform your life and find joy and happiness in all that you do. Sound too good to be true? It's not…it's very possible. All I ask of you is for you to be aware and mindful. Open up and listen. Breathe. Focus intently on what I'm trying to say to you. Focus on what I'm writing. If you do, you will feel and see amazing results in your life and the lives that surround you.

Life is a wonderful thing. Each day can be beautiful. Every day can be happy. Be grateful. It's all up to you. Live in the Present. Embrace your current life with enthusiasm and compassion. Yes, you have to work at it and take action. Finding optimum health takes action. Losing weight takes work. It takes willpower and discipline. It takes a strong and focused mind and spirit. You need to feel the joy of this everyday…get into the experience of transformation and growth. Get excited about it! This is part of your strategy towards success and change.

These days more and more of us have our own individual spirituality. Many of us practice what is called "practical spirituality", that is day-to-day spirituality in action. Whether it is at home or work, with friends, family, co-workers or strangers, many people are trying to adapt their spiritual lives into their day-to-day experiences.

I firmly believe you have to have faith in something larger than yourself. We are all connected. The mystery of it all is the exciting part. That is part of the journey.

My book is organized into two sections. The first is a general philosophy and discussion of health - physical, mental, spiritual and emotional. I have divided it into 25 short chapters so they are easy to read if you have limited time. I want you to reread the various chapters individually from time-to-time to remind yourself of some important principles. The name of the chapter itself is a reference to a principle or guideline, so focus on that thought. I suggest you read a chapter, then take some time to think and absorb that principle. I have questions at the end of each chapter; use those to guide you if you wish. These guidelines are very important for your success in health and weight loss, so please include them in your overall plan.

At the end of the first section I have also put together several summary worksheets of powerful statements on success, affirmations, general facts about attitude and the power of thought. A special section on the 'Power of Attraction" also gives you some great guidelines towards success and a happier life. Use these daily to help you with your program. Pick some of your favorite thoughts and affirmations and make up your own goal and vision statement. Remember the law of attraction states "what you think and feel manifests", therefore it is essential to tune your body, mind, spirit and emotions into your vision of success and overall health.

My second section focuses on the <u>*Natural Health &*</u>
<u>*Weight Loss Program*</u>. This is a specific step-by-step
program in which you can follow to get on the right track
for health & weight loss. If you believe and make the
effort, it will change your life as it did mine.
I guarantee it!

My overall program is about changing the mind and
heart as much as the body. Learning to work with all
parts of ourselves for optimum health is the key. When
you tune into yourself, when you tune into the energy
field that is all around us, when you tune into the body,
mind, spirit and emotions and allow them to work for
you, you will see amazing changes.

Remember your body is your shell, your biological
cover. There is something much grander than that…and
this is your spirit. Losing weight and becoming healthy
is about attitude and belief as much as it is about exercise
and diet. You need all of these elements to succeed.
When you learn to honor and love your inner self and
tune in to the greater universe you will gain the strength
and understanding to do anything.

I'm very excited for you. My life has changed
dramatically and I want yours to also change. I want you
to connect with the Universe and feel the vibrant energy
and health that we all can have.

Section I -
The Connection Between
Body, Mind, Spirit & Emotions

1 - *The Dark Night of the Soul*

Pain and depression is not a fun experience, yet it also can be an important tool for change and transformation. This is the body and mind telling you something. Telling you that something is out of balance and needs to be changed. The term "dark night of the soul" comes from a book of that same name by St. John of the Cross. As a religious man St. John went through a spiritual crisis before he saw the light. Most anyone of importance and fame, including all of our avatars and religious icons, have gone through a major life crisis, a depression or a stressful event. This event or mood caused them to look deep within to find the answers. And what they found was their inner strength, their connection with the divine source. Through this crisis they rose from the negative depths to beauty and joy. Barbara Brennan in her great book *Hands of Light* sums it up "Pain teaches us to ask for help and healing and is, therefore, a key to education of the soul." Hard times build character and strength. The Dalai Lama in his book *How to Practice the Way of a Meaningful Life* writes, "Hard times build determination and inner strength...trying circumstances provide us with invaluable opportunities to practice tolerance and patience."

If you are having a crisis or depression try to look inward and find your strength. Do not let it consume you. Let the negative feelings give you hope. Take time to really analyze why you are feeling that way.

Is it time for a change? What do you need to do to improve your life? Ask for help from the universe and let it go. Have faith that you will get some answers. Listen to your intuition. And most of all try to reach for a higher more positive feeling. Get yourself out of the depression, or the anger or guilt or stress. Start focusing on being grateful. Seek help if you need to, but know that you are in control of how you think and feel.

1-Summary Questions & Guidelines –

1. Is there a lesson that you are learning with this negative experience?

2. Is there a chance for growth or change?

3. Try to find a positive reason(s) for your pain. Focus on that.

2- *How We Weave Tales of Woe and Sadness*

Why do humans suffer? Why do we focus on the tales of sadness? Do you know if we learned to focus on the positive, on not letting hardship get to you, that your life would be better? Happiness is a state of being. So is Sadness. One feels good, the other not so good. Which would you prefer? The more we focus on sadness and suffering the more it consumes us. We can take a step forward and acknowledge suffering, show compassion, but not let it take control of us. Depression is a low frequency emotion…sadness takes you away from the higher vibrations of love and happiness. It is good to feel sadness over another's suffering…empathy and sympathy are good attributes in a person. But when sadness takes over your emotional state for a long period of time this is not healthy. When you focus on the "poor me" attitude, it only brings that emotional state to you. You do not become happy or successful when you are sad, so why would you want to be? Why do you want to dwell on misery and woe when you can be happy and joyful instead? When you feed into sadness and depression you get more of the same. When you let it go and work on being positive, you attract this into your life.

Life can be very difficult. The path is not always easy. Yet when you can shift your attitude from negative to positive, from sadness to happiness, you feel much better. Start today to shift your thinking.

When you feel sorry for yourself or dwell on the negative, acknowledge that, and then re-direct your thoughts to the positive. As you do this more and more you will notice a change in yourself.

2-Summary Questions & Guidelines –

1. Try to find the reason behind your depression or sadness. Take some time to really think about it.

2. What is at the core of it all?

3. Can you change your emotions and feelings to a more positive state?

3- *You Cannot Avoid Change*

Change is constant. Things are in a constant state of flux. Every day is different. We are not the same person yesterday as we are today. Neither are friends or family. When you accept this fact your life will be easier. Caroline Myss sums it up in her great book <u>*Anatomy of the Spirit*</u> ,"Consciousness is the ability to release the old and embrace the new…this truth is difficult to learn to live with because human beings seek stability – the absence of change. Therefore becoming conscious means living fully in the present moment, knowing that no situation or person will be exactly the same tomorrow." So we have a choice to accept change and "go with the flow" of life or we can resist change and seek stability. Which do you prefer? When you can embrace change your stress level goes way down. When you can just accept that life is about constant growth and change, death and rebirth, it is easier to just accept changes and not get angry or upset. Learn to just let go of many of the daily surprises that unfold. If we allow it, little things can affect our moods for the entire day. Instead just laugh about it. Brush it off. Accept it and move on. The more excited you can get about change and the less stress it causes you, the better your life will be. Embrace the constant change of life.

3-Summary Questions & Guidelines –

1. Do not resist change. When it comes to you just let it go.

2. Can you view change as a positive thing?

3. Can you get excited and enthusiastic about change?

4- The Connection of Mind, Body, Spirit and Emotion

These four parts of ourselves are connected. You can't have one without the other. You can, but you will be out of harmony and balance. Ancient traditions, including our European and Eastern ancestors, focused on the connection of Earth, Air, Water and Fire, the four elements. The wheel or circle was a sacred symbol for it showed the interrelation of all four elements. The medicine wheel was and still is an important symbol of the connection between the four elements. Each element was identified with a part of yourself. In most indigenous cultures, Earth represents the Body, Air represents the Mind, Fire represents Spirit and Water represents Emotions. This exact match was not exclusive to all traditions, but in general all indigenous cultures utilize this same idea and practice; that of harmony between the four parts of ourselves. When one was out of balance or out of harmony with another you had illness or disease. This is true of us today. For example, when you have a sound body, but your emotions are not in a healthy state you are out of harmony with source energy. You must work on all four elements to be healthy.

There is one more element I will mention here, we have already mentioned it and we will discuss it again in the other chapters….this is what we call Ether or the Universal Spirit, Source Energy, the Universal Energy Field, or to some God. Keep that element in mind also as it connects all parts of our self to the larger energy world. This is also an essential element to be in connection with. The more you are in harmony with your body, mind, spirit and emotions, the more you are in harmony with source energy.

Do not forget any part of yourself. Nurture each one. Evaluate the needs of each one. Know that your success in overall health and weight loss combines all four of these elements working together in harmony.

4-Summary Questions & Guidelines –

1. Are the four parts of you in harmony?

2. What can you do to improve this harmony?

3. Which part needs the most work?

5- *Religion and Spirituality*

Many people get a bit confused over the difference between religion and spirituality. And many that do know the difference do not find fulfillment out of a particular religion, yet consider themselves spiritual. Eckhart Tolle helps us understand the difference in <u>The New Earth</u> "Many people are already aware of the difference between spirituality and religion. They realize that having a belief system – a set of thoughts that you regard as the absolute truth-does not make you spiritual no matter what the nature of those beliefs is. In fact, the more you make your beliefs into your identity, the more cut off you are from the spiritual dimension within yourself." Being spiritual he says "…has nothing to do with what you believe, but everything to do with your state of consciousness. This in turn, determines how you act in the world and interact with others." Where do you fit in this picture? Do you feel that you are spiritual, but do not connect with any particular religion? Or do you have a religion, but are trying to find some deeper meaning out of the teachings? You are not alone.

Millions of people, in particular the younger generations, are seeking more spiritual meaning in their lives. A new movement that is gaining momentum is what many call "practical spirituality". This is what I utilize in my program. It is an awareness, a consciousness of a higher energy source that we are all connected to. This energy source can be called many things, that is not important. What is important is that you have a belief and faith in something larger than you; something that is you, but more that you; something that we are all connected to and all of us have access to. Isn't this a great concept?

If you are more of a scientist you can research quantum-physics and see that everything is energy. That we all come from the Zero Point Field and we are connected to this energy. Spirituality also acknowledges this connection. Albert Einstein sums up the connection of spirituality and science, "I maintain that cosmic religious feeling is the strongest and noblest incitement to scientific research." So even if you have a difficult time being "spiritual" realize that we are all connected to a higher energy source. And for many of us we acknowledge this fact and it becomes part of our awareness and spirituality.

5-Summary Questions & Guidelines –

1. Do you consider yourself religious?

2. Do you consider yourself spiritual?

3. What are your beliefs? Can you write them down or explain them to someone?

4. Do you believe in a higher power or higher energy?

6- *The Power of Thought*

Your thoughts are very powerful. They are the basis of your reality. Your thoughts and feelings manifest your reality. As Ramtha states in his book *The White Book* "All of your tomorrows are designed by your thoughts this very day." Thoughts and feelings are the ultimate creators. This is one of the secrets that you need to embrace. Remember an affirmative thought is 100 times more powerful than a negative thought. When you think positive you are affecting your body and spirit. You are inviting positive energy to you, your body loves this. If you affirm negative thoughts you will attract them. When you focus on negative attitudes you will attract negativity. Negative thoughts such as fear, depression, anger, envy, etc. cause stress and lower your overall energy. Anger affects your consciousness and everyone around you. As Ramtha states again "Every thought in your mind is true, for it is alive in consciousness." Barbara Brennan writes "Thoughts and emotions move between people in time and space through the human energy field."

I must remind you that you are in control of your thoughts. This is another important secret you should remember. You are the only one who creates your reality. Simple change of thoughts and words can instantly change your mood and the energy that surrounds you. All circumstance can be changed in a moment.

William James, the father of modern psychology claims that a person can change the quality of their life by changing the quality of their thoughts. This is where you need to grasp this important connection. Do not give your power away. Be aware of your thoughts as they happen. Alter your thoughts when necessary to help obtain your goals of health, happiness and weight loss.

6-Summary Questions & Guidelines –

1. Are you able to control your thoughts?

2. What kinds of thoughts dominate your thinking?

3. Are you able to think in a positive way?

4. Can you shift your thinking and be aware of your thoughts and feelings?

7 – *The Law of Attraction*

This is the other big secret. Thought attracts like a magnet. The images you hold in your mind attract similar images and experiences. Whatever feeling you are thinking you tend to attract the most. This is a basic principle everyone should know and attempt to follow. Abraham and Esther Hicks in the book *Ask and it is Given* explain "Every thought vibrates, every thought radiates a signal, and every thought attracts a matching signal back. We call that process the Law of Attraction…by the Powerful Universal Law of Attraction, you draw to you the essence of whatever you are predominantly thinking about." This principle is pretty straightforward and in my opinion guides the universe. It is a key to your success in health and weight loss and in life. What you think and feel manifests. Now this does not happen instantly, but with focus, intention, desire, and action it does eventually make itself clear to you. Think about it, when you are positive and happy, you usually attract that type of energy or experience around you. In the very least negative things do not bother you. When you are negative, angry, depressed, fearful, etc. you tend to attract that type of energy or experience. Has this not happened to you? Elizabeth Towne states in the classic book *The Life Power & How to Use It*, "Man is a magnet, and every line and dot and detail of his experiences come by his own attraction." If you are not familiar with the Law of Attraction I highly recommend *Ask and It is Given* and the DVD or Book

The Secret. They will explain this law very thoroughly.

Remember one other important thing. It is our emotions and feelings that guide us with this law. So it is thought with feeling that manifests reality. Your feeling is what Abraham calls your "Emotional Guidance System". This system allows you to attract more positive energy and experiences. See the emotional scale chart at the end of this section for an idea as to where most emotions fit. Most of all focus on feelings of appreciation, gratitude, joy, freedom and love. When you focus on these things you are manifesting powerful source energy that will help you in all that you do.

7-Summary Questions & Guidelines –

1. What thought and emotion do you focus on the most?

2. Are you able to change your thoughts and feelings from negative to positive?

3. Are you a positive person?

4. What type of energy do you attract?

8 – Start the Revolution Within

This is the title of my book and appropriately so. Humans are known to look on the outside for the answers. We try so hard to change our external circumstances to make things better and to make us happier. "If only I had a better house", "If only I had a better body", "If only I had more money". Sound familiar? These recordings play again and again in most of our minds. We are fortunate that there has been a strong movement towards the Eastern religious practices. That has helped us re-introduce ourselves to practices that focus on the inward journey-which one must start with changing their inner self before they can change anything else. Many revolutions have started on the outside, but we are at a time where the true awakening for humans and our planet is a focus on the inner journey. This inner awakening is what all of our religious teachers have been telling us for centuries-that to seek God or the Universe or Source Energy you seek it from within. Our true essence is our spirit and soul. This connects us to the universe, to the universal energy field. We first must go inward to connect with source energy. Meditation is one way to do this. We must evaluate our unconscious or subconscious beliefs and patterns. Hypnotherapy and other techniques such as those are a great way to go inward and deal with this part of you.

Whatever you do it is essential that you work on your inner being. You need to erase those old recordings, those old thoughts and beliefs, and install new values that attract health and happiness. The revolution begins within.

8- *Summary Questions & Guidelines* –

1. Do you have old recordings and beliefs that need to be erased?

2. Are you aware of your beliefs and how they control your thoughts?

3. Do you meditate and spend time focusing on your inner being or subconscious?

4. Are there beliefs that you would like to change?

5. Are there beliefs that hold you back from your true desires and goals?

9- *The Act of Giving*

To give is to receive. Deepak Chopra in his book <u>*The Seven Spiritual Laws of Success*</u> makes it evident as to the importance of giving, "The universe operates through dynamic exchange…giving and receiving are different aspects of the flow of energy in the universe. And in our willingness to give that which we seek, we keep the abundance of the universe circulating in our lives."

When we give we need to give freely without expectations. This can be a difficult task to some. The gift of giving is enough. And the universe will respond to that energy of giving…it will return to you in some form. In a world of "what's in it for me", it is essential that we reverse that trend and become givers unconditionally. I am not talking about giving away your power or your freedom. I am talking about simple gifts of love, appreciation and compassion. Making someone happy with a compliment, or a prayer or flower. Helping someone without them asking. Simple gifts of giving go along way. And the gift of giving radiates to everyone who is involved. It alters the energy field in a positive manner. If we think about the law of attraction and apply it to this concept we understand the importance of giving on an energy level. When you smile at a stranger you are giving out energy. You are a giver and this is a good thing. Practice this as often as you can and you will see results of a better life.

9- Summary Questions & Guidelines –

1. Do you give to others on a regular basis?

2. Do you give freely without expecting anything in return?

3. How do you feel when you give?

10- Fear, Depression, Anger, Judgment & Low Frequency Emotions

Low frequency emotions are emotions that do not connect us with the higher energy field in a positive way. They are usually "hurtful" emotions. They tend to hurt others and hurt ourselves. The top low frequency emotions are fear, depression, despair, grief, regret, jealousy, hatred, rage, anger, and revenge. All of these emotions and feelings illicit what many call "bad vibes". They are not good for you or for others. They do not help manifest positive experiences in your life. The more you can avoid these negative emotions the better it is for your health and life. If you tend to be in this negative state most of the time, it's time for a change. It is said that negative emotions cause illness and disease. They are simply not healthy or beneficial. We all feel these from time-to-time. Instead of feeling "guilty" (one of the negative emotions by the way) we need to recognize the feeling and let it go. It is important we then move on to another more positive feeling. Eckhart Tolle writes in *The New Earth*, "Fear, anxiety, expectation, regret, guilt, anger are all dysfunctions of the time-bound state of consciousness. Time is the ego's friend." When we operate from ego alone we tend to be self-centered in a negative way. Depression is a self-centered tendency as one is absorbed in the misery and sadness of life. This is why it is a low frequency emotion. It is the opposite of happiness and joy. What would you rather experience?

10-Summary Questions & Guidelines –

1. What emotions are in your life?

2. Do you focus on lower frequency emotions?

3. Are you able to shift your thoughts and feelings to higher frequency positive emotions?

11- Get Clear on what you Want!

Socrates once said "The unexamined life is not worth living." It is very important to get clear on what you want in life. Want to be healthy and lose weight? Get clear on this goal and vision. Focus on what you will achieve, not what you don't have. James Ray in <u>Harmonic Wealth</u> writes, "Get crystal clear about what you want-see it in 3D. See it, feel it, smell it, taste it, hear it, and make it specific and measurable…ramp up those feelings, take action every day." Joe Vitale in <u>Attractor Factor</u> also emphasis the importance of focusing on what you want in a positive way, not what you don't want. "How do you know if you're clear right now? Think of something that you want to have, do or be. Why don't you have it yet? If your answer is something negative, you aren't clear."

What do you want? If it's health and weight loss that is your focus, get clear on where you see yourself. How many pounds do you want to lose? Can you see yourself feeling great? Can you see and feel it? Do you have a plan of action? It is essential when we want something that we focus on positive intent. We focus our vision on achieving it, not on where we are now. And it is essential that you do not focus on the negative of not having it. You need to allow the universe to pick up on your intent and desire. Most of all you need to be positive and visualize yourself as already having achieved the goal. This will set everything else in motion.

11- Summary Questions & Guidelines –

1. Where are your thoughts and actions?

2. Where is your conversation and focus?

3. Are you clear? Are there any negative beliefs that are holding you back?

12 – When We Heal Ourselves, We Heal Others

We first must work on ourselves before we try to work on others. Our first and foremost task is to be selfish and heal ourselves. The famous ancient Greek saying "Know Thyself" still rings true in the modern age. We cannot focus on the externals until we do the internal work. Buddhists and other Eastern religions have practiced the inward journey for centuries. Meditation is one way to go inward and heal ourselves.

We have an effect on everyone around us. If we have negative emotions such as depression or anger, we are not doing anyone good. To heal these negative emotions we must journey inward to our spirit and unconsciousness. We need to look at our beliefs and life patterns. This is a time to possibly seek help from a healer or counselor. Someone who can help you with the inward journey. Do not think that going to someone makes you a "failure"…it is exactly the opposite. You are wise and strong by seeking some assistance. This is also a great time to start a meditation practice! In reality we cannot heal others, they have to heal themselves. We can guide and teach others, but to do so we have to be strong. We have to know our own power and be connected to source energy and to the universe. This is an inward journey.

12-Summary Questions & Guidelines –

1. Do you meditate? Are you willing to try?

2. Have you ever gone to a counselor?

3. What are your beliefs? Are there some of them that are holding you back from your full potential?

13 – *Nature for Inspiration*

Nature is our best teacher. Go outside as much as you can and be part of nature and the earth. Go for walks. Sit by a stream or in a forest. Go camping or for a hike. Be still and silent. Listen to the wind or water. Listen to your inner voice within the stillness of nature. Nature is there to remind you of the beauty of the universe. It is here to inspire and nurture you.

For indigenous cultures the relation and responsibility to Nature and to all creation is an essential part of their belief. Sun Bear in his book <u>*Dancing with the Wheel*</u> writes, "In the Native teachings we acknowledge that all parts of the creation are our relations because we live on the same Earth Mother and get water, air, food, fuel and shelter from her. We are all related. The Earth needs more of her children to take their rightful position as her keepers. To do this we must have an ever-increasing commitment to the earth and an ever-growing understanding of her needs."

We rely on Nature for life. But remember it gives us much more than food, shelter and fuel. It reminds us of the harmony in the universe. It inspires us to be compassionate. It gives us the connection to pure potentiality. When you sit and commune with nature you are talking to the spirit of the universe. You are seeing and feeling firsthand the sacredness of all life and energy.

Remember Nature can help you become realigned with life; it can help you see and feel a higher order and purpose. Get out into Nature as often as you can to heal and get inspired.

13-Summary Questions & Guidelines –

1. Do you go into Nature often?

2. When you are in Nature do you take time to be silent and still?

3. Do you relate to our connection to Nature and the Earth?

14 – Happiness is the Fuel of Success

Happiness and Joy are the magic lubricant of success. They are among the highest emotional frequencies that we can achieve. Pure Joy and Happiness give us unlimited power. Pure Joy and Happiness allow us to connect with source energy on the most active level. When we do so we activate a positive attraction to great things in our lives. If there is one thing we can do to help our lives it would to be in a state of happiness. And happiness and joy is equal to love. Neal Donald Walsch in his inspiring book *Conversations with God-Book 1* dictates from his connection to God or Source Energy, "What the soul is after is-the highest feeling of love you can imagine. This is the purpose...the highest feeling is to experience the unity with all that is." So if the universe is telling us to strive for love then this is the ultimate energy and purpose. Many authors, teachers, scientists and successful business people are saying the same thing-that to be happy, to feel love and joy is the ultimate connection to the universe. That this connection will bring us great success with our intents and desires. Now even on a more "logical" level, to be happy and to give or feel love makes you in a better mood. And this mood usually makes others happy around you. And it also creates the energy of happiness. People tend to be more successful and productive when they are happy. When you "spread the love" so-to-speak you are benefiting yourself in many obvious ways.

To sum up my feelings on the power of love, Marc Allen in his wonderful book *The Greatest Secret of All* writes, "We know the secret, deep in our hearts. We've always known the secret. To love one another, and all of creation, is the greatest secret of all. Love overcomes fear, and transforms our lives and our world."

14-Summary Questions & Guidelines –

1. Are you able to keep in a happy or joyful state of mind?

2. Are you comfortable being loving and kind towards others?

3. Do you hold back love, joy and happiness?

4. Does it make you comfortable? Or uncomfortable?

15 – Live in the Moment

Eckhart Tolle and Deepak Chopra among many great writers and teachers teach us to be in the Moment, to be in the Present. When we focus our energies on the Now, on the Present, we are most attached to the Divine, to Source Energy and the Universe. When we are distracted with thoughts of the past or future, our energy is not there. It gets diffused and filtered through our belief systems and what Eckhart Tolle calls our "Pain-Body". Learn to become attentive to your thoughts. Be aware of your negative thoughts as they happen. We carry around a burden of our past that controls our lives. The "Pain-Body" theory states that we hold negative past emotions and experiences in our minds and bodies. These make up our ego and influence how we live, act and feel. Blaming others for our problems is a big part of this. We limit ourselves through regret, hostility and guilt. Yet none of this controls us. We can break free from the past and return to our place of Power-that is the Present. Let go of expectations and stop identifying with your pain-body, with your past. Let go of the "story" and create your "reality" in the present. Learn to let go and accept all events and situations as a learning experience. Be present when you are listening to others. Try not to think about your response before they are done talking. Just being aware that your thoughts, feelings and actions will help you take control and connect with you to the Present and with the Divine.

By being Present, by living in the moment, your life will improve in many great ways. And in times of stress just remember the famous phrase "This too shall pass."

15-Summary Questions & Guidelines –

1. Where are your thoughts right now?

2. How much time did you spend today focusing on the past? On the future?

3. Try to focus on the Present for a few minutes. How does it feel? Try this every day and see if it helps you.

16 - Breathing & Stillness

Thich Nhat Hanh in <u>*Peace is Every Step*</u> writes, "While we practice conscious breathing, our thinking will slow down, and we give ourselves a real rest. Most of the time, we think too much, and mindful breathing helps us to be calm, relaxed, and peaceful." Breathing helps you slow down and focus. It is what many call a doorway to access your spirit and the universe. Stillness creates space between thoughts and feelings. Work on creating gaps and space between your constant thinking.

Buddhism and most Eastern religions focus much time on breathing and meditation. Conscious breath taken several times a day is a great way to bring mindfulness and presence into your life. Breathing helps you focus on the present…it brings you to the moment. The Dalai Lama gives us some pointers about breathing and meditation, "Do not let your mind think on what has happened in the past, nor let it chase after things that might happen in the future; rather leave the mind vivid, without any constructions, just as it is." What he is describing is being present and mindful. Letting go of any past or future distractions.

When you breathe, breathe slowly, in and out. Do this several times letting go with the out breath. Focus on your breathing and let go of any thoughts you may have. Be gentle, don't force out the thoughts, just let go of them slowly. For help focus on the words "in" and "out" as you synchronize your breathing. Or focus on another spiritual object or symbol, anything that keeps you mindful of your breathing. When you only have a spare moment, just take a bit of time to breathe in and out a few times. When you are stressed or angry, utilize the same technique. Taking time to breathe is essential to your overall health.

16-Summary Questions & Guidelines –

1. Do you focus any time on just breathing?

2. Do you meditate or have quiet time?

3. Can you dedicate some time each day to focus on mindful breathing?

17 - Practice Mindfulness

Mindfulness is being aware of your thoughts, feelings and actions, how they affect you, and how they affect others. It is being "mindful" of what you say to others before you say it. It is awareness of the universal energy field and how we are all connected to it. As we discussed in the last chapter breathing and meditation helps you focus on being mindful. Mindfulness is a state of mind that you learn. It is an awareness. A consciousness. When you are aware of your actions towards yourself and others and can step back and view them, you are being mindful.

Thich Nhat Hanh in *Being Peace* tells us about the mindfulness vows he teaches, "I vow to develop my compassion in order to love and protect the life of people, animals, plants and minerals. I vow to develop understanding in order to be able to love and to live in harmony with people, plants, animals and minerals." This is the focus of mindfulness. And you notice also how mindfulness is focusing on things beyond people. This is the essence of being mindful. Being aware of all relations and all things in our world and universe. Ask yourself "Am I being mindful?" each time you have to make a decision. Use breathing and meditation to make a big decision. And take some time to focus and let it go to the universe. After some practice this will come naturally. It can be learned.

17-Summary Questions & Guidelines –

1. Do you practice mindfulness?

2. Are you aware of your thoughts, feelings and actions?

3. Are you able to step back and see a situation without reacting?

18 - Law of Detachment - Let Go!

Detachment is a strong Buddhist concept and is becoming better known in modern Western thinking also. It is the art of letting go and allowing. Deepak Chopra in *The Seven Spiritual Laws of Success* writes, "In detachment lies the wisdom of uncertainty. In the wisdom of uncertainty lies freedom from our past, from the known, which is the prison of past conditioning. And in our willingness to step into the unknown…we surrender ourselves to the creative mind that orchestrates the dance of the universe."

Detachment allows us the freedom to not be judgmental. To allow oneself and those around us the freedom to be as they are. Detachment also allows us to Let Go, to allow energy and circumstance to just flow. This allows the universe to manifest our goals and visions. If we are so wound up and stressed over our desires we are actually attracting that negative energy. When you learn to relax and let go it changes everything. Now letting go isn't the same as sitting around and being lazy. It means not expecting an anticipated outcome. It means letting go of controlling people and circumstances. As Caroline Myss in *Anatomy of the Spirit* writes, "Detachment does not mean ceasing to care. It means stilling one's fear-driven voices." When we let go of the fear and step into the possibilities with excitement it opens us and the universe up to true potential. Learn to let go.

18-Summary Questions & Guidelines –

1. Are you able to detach from an expected outcome?

2. Do you like to control situations and others?

3. Are you able to get excited about the uncertainty of an event or circumstance? Can you learn?

19 - We are Made of Water

Did you know we were mostly made of water? Some say over 70% of our body is water. Water is a great conductor of energy and therefore is subject to energy manipulation. A great experiment was done by Dr Masura Emoto with his book *The Hidden Messages in Water*. In it he photographed molecules of water that had been subject to positive and negative messages in various ways, including pure spring water and polluted water. In one experiment he attached written notes attached to bottles of water. The negative messages were messages like "You make me sick, I will kill you.", the positive messages were "love" and "thank you". Now get this…these were messages placed on the bottles of water. Contrary to the prevailing wisdom of science the water responded to these messages. Under a microscope, the water with the positive messages formed beautiful crystals while the water with the negative messages became ugly and malformed. What does that mean to us?

We have to remember that we are all connected with water. Our planet is mostly water as is our body. The interesting thing is if thoughts can do that to water what can they do to us? And what about our bodies? If we pollute our bodies with chemicals and negative thoughts how is our energy affected? How does our water look under a microscope?

19-Summary Questions & Guidelines –

1. How clean is the water inside you?

2. How much clean water do you drink daily?

3. What are your thoughts and feelings doing to your body?

20- The Power of Emotion and Feelings

Emotion and Feelings are powerful. As Joe Vitale writes in *The Attractor Factor*, "Emotion has power. Emotion also has the power to create what you want….the energy in the emotion will work to pull you toward the thing you want while also pulling the thing you want towards you." Want health and weight loss? Attract it by your thoughts and feelings. Listen to your feelings and intuitions as they are designed to help you.

Positive emotions guide you towards alignment with the universe. Bob Proctor in his book *You Were Born Rich* writes, "Learn to follow the quiet voice within that speaks in feelings rather than words; follow what you 'hear' inside, rather than what others may be telling you to do." Abraham and Esther Hicks in *Ask and it is Given* stress the importance of emotions in all your decisions. Our lives are affected by our emotions. They are in what Esther Hicks and Abraham say is our "guidance system". What you think and feel manifests. A simple shift of emotions can change your day. Whatever you are feeling is a perfect reflection of what is in the process of becoming. Bad vibes and negative emotions are telling you something. Positive emotions align you with the universe, with source energy. Learn to focus on positive emotions and feelings.

20-Summary Questions & Guidelines –

1. What emotions do you focus on the most?

2. Do you experience positive or negative emotions the most?

3. Can you change and focus on positive emotions and feelings?

21 - Your Body Cells & Energy

Day-to-Day fearful or bitter attitudes are biologically negative substances. According to energy medicine we are living history books. Our bodies contain our histories. Think of an illness as a power disorder. What drains your spirit also drains your body. As Caroline Myss states in her book *Anatomy of the Spirit* ," If a person's spirit is impelled by Fear, then Fear returns to her energy field and to her body. If she directs her spirit in faith, however, then grace returns to her energy field and her biological system thrives." Scientist and healer Barbara Brennan believes that our cell tissues hold the vibrational patterns of our attitudes and our belief systems. Positive and negative experiences register a memory in cell tissue as well as in the energy field at large. Her theories are backed up by science.

Remember that all of our thoughts and feelings enter our system as energy. When it is positive energy it helps the system. When it is negative energy it hurts the system. Many holistic doctors and scientists believe there is one thing that causes Illness and Disease – Stress. Stress is brought on by negative emotions and feelings.
Day-to-day fearful, negative or bitter attitudes are negative substances. Our "memory" of experiences is stored in our body tissue.

So what can we do about this? It's fairly simple…think and feel positive. Get rid of negative emotions as they occur. A positive thought, emotion and feeling is much more powerful than a negative one, so by default once you train your mind to be positive your body will begin to respond to this signal. This is another secret of health, happiness and weight loss.

21-Summary Questions & Guidelines –

1. Where are your thoughts and feelings most of the time?

2. Do you focus on the negative? Are you stressed?

3. Can you refocus your thoughts and feelings?

4. Can you learn to be positive?

22 -*Visualize the Life you Want*

Visualizing your goals and desires is a key to change and success. Without the internal vision of what you want to be, your chances of success are lessoned. Great athletes use visualization techniques to improve their performance. Science shows us that the mind does not distinguish between when you visualize and when you actually perform the action. The same brain chemicals and neurons fire up. Therefore visualizing your goals is very important. It is important to remember to think and feel what you desire. If you desire weight loss, you need to visualize your ideal weight. And then you need to feel the success of it, the joy. Doesn't it feel great? You want to feel this happiness. Don't feel uncomfortable about it. You are setting the energy in motion. You are tuning up your mind, spirit and emotions…the body will soon follow. When your mind and spirit are convinced of your intent through visualization, your body chemistry will start to transform. This is another of the secrets of health and permanent weight loss.

Now I stress again that you have to work at it also. You have to actualize your goals. Sitting in front of the TV eating potato chips won't change your weight no matter how hard you visualize. What visualization does though is help you get into action. It gives you that positive energy and motivation to do so. And it puts source energy and the universe on your side! You attract a positive outcome by being positive.

James Ray in <u>*Harmonic Wealth*</u> sums it up, "Great achievers focus only on their visions and fire those visions with wisdom, courage and commitment, regardless of their current circumstance. They know it's only a matter of time before their visions come into physical form." It is very important to focus on your visions and be patient in their manifestation.

I have included a worksheet at the end of this section to help you with visualization. Make sure it is part of your daily schedule.

22-Summary Questions & Guidelines –

1. Do you know how to visualize? Learn the techniques.

2. When you visualize do you see your intended outcome and your future?

3. Do you use your emotions and feelings?

4. Are you visualizing success on a daily basis?

23- Resistance is What Holds us Back

When we resist change and resist following our heart and intuition we usually struggle. Fear is resistance. Anger is resistance. Depression is resistance. The more you can open up to the Universe and learn to let go, the more you will attract great things into your life! The great psychologist Carl Jung says "what you resist persists" …meaning as long as we focus on the negative, on what we don't want, we will attract that energy and not obtain freedom and joy. And freedom and joy are keys to your success. They say resistance is what holds us back. It's what keeps us from the full benefit of Source Energy, and of the Divine. You and your feelings are all that is responsible for whether you let in your Well-being or not. As Abraham and Esther Hicks say "There is only a stream of Well-being that flows. You can allow it or you can resist it, but it flows just the same." This "flow" is Source Energy. This is the energy of the Universe. It is here to help you succeed and be happy.

If your goal is to be healthy than you need to let go of all resistance and ask the universe to assist you. The higher vibration emotions such as love, joy, happiness, enthusiasm, appreciation, gratitude, passion and eagerness are the fuel of your success in achieving your goals. A positive attitude and belief is the key. Let go of any resistance and you will see a great change in yourself.

23-*Summary Questions & Guidelines* –

1. What is your main Resistance? Fear? Depression? Jealousy? Anger? Guilt?

2. How often do you focus on these feelings?

3. Are you able to change these feeling to the positive emotions?

4. What happens when you do?

24- The Ripple Effect

The Ripple Effect is a well known idea. I will explain it in two ways as an analogy.

1.) You are a rock with energy. When the rock is thrown into the "water of life" you immediately splash and ripples wake outward from your energy. Now think about this. As a human, your energy ripples outwards to affect everything around you. When it is a positive ripple it affects people and things in a positive way. When it is negative it affects people in that way. Either way there is a ripple. The ripple is energy.

2.) Let's take another water example. When you see a river or stream there are usually rapids of some kind. What causes the rapids? The cause is the rocks or log or terrain before the actual rapid. Again, you are the rock or log. The water is the energy of life. It passes over you and you affect it. You affect the future with your energy as the water is carried downstream.

The whole point of both of these analogies is that we affect people and things with our energy. Whether it is positive, such as joy, happiness or enthusiasm, or negative, such as anger, jealousy or depression, you still affect those around you. Which energies do you want to give out?

24- Summary Questions & Guidelines –

1. What kind of ripples are you sending outward?

2. Can you change your ripples from negative to positive?

3. How do people around you relate to your energy?

25- *Create your Reality Every Day.*

You are in control of your life. You create your reality. It is essential every day that you create your reality. You can change your thoughts and emotions. Through positive affirmations, visualization, prayer and meditation you can connect with your higher power and source energy. Start each day with gratitude for the day, for what you have. Give thanks for what you have, and what you desire. Make your desires into present tense. See my summary worksheet on affirmations and visualization to help you with this. The universe loves positive intent!

Dr Joe Dispenza in the book and movie *What the BLEEP do We know!?* summarizes the idea of creating your reality every day, "I wake up in the morning and I consciously create my day the way I want it to happen… When I create my day and out of nowhere little things happen that are so unexplainable, I know that they are the process or the result of my creation. And the more I do that, the more I build a neural net in my brain that I accept that that's possible…So if we're consciously designing our destiny, and if we're consciously from a spiritual standpoint throwing in with the idea that our thoughts can affect our reality or affect our life -- because reality equals life -- then I have this little pact that I have when I create my day. I say, I'm taking this time to create my day and I'm infecting the quantum field…. And as I do that during parts of the day, I'll have thoughts that are so amazing, that cause a chill in my physical body that have come from nowhere. But then I remember that that thought has an associated energy that's produced an effect in my physical body. Now that's a subjective experience, but the truth is I don't think that unless I was creating my day to have unlimited thought, that that thought would come."

Take time each day to create your reality. This is done through visualization, affirmations and meditation.

25-Summary Questions & Guidelines –

1. Do you have time in the morning to create your day?

2. Can you visualize your day and create a positive future?

3. Can you make this part of your daily routine?

Section I – Summary Worksheets

1. *Scale of your Emotions*

2. *Your Body and its Connection to Mind, Spirit & Emotions*

3. *The Power of Thought and the Law of Attraction*

4. *Steps towards Utilizing the Law of Attraction & Being Present*

5. *A Few Positive Concepts to Live By*

6. *Notes on Visualization, Affirmations, Meditation & Goals/Visions -*

Scale of your Emotions

Below is a summary developed by Abraham, Esther and Jerry Hicks in their wonderful book about the Law of Attraction *Ask and It Is Given*. I highly recommend it.

The scale is a list of the highest & most positive emotions to connect with, going down to the lowest and most negative. This gives you an idea as to where certain emotions lie in the scale. This list is, of course, not a rule, but a guideline. The goal is to always strive for the higher frequency emotions and avoid the lower frequency ones. If you can stay with the top 7 as much as possible and avoid the bottom 8 you will see positive life change in many ways. Be aware daily of where you are on the scale. Give it a try.

1. Joy/Knowledge /Freedom/Love/Appreciation
2. Passion
3. Enthusiasm/Eagerness/Happiness
4. Positive Expectation/Belief
5. Optimism
6. Hopefulness
7. Contentment
8. Boredom
9. Pessimism
10. Frustration/Irritation/Impatience
11. "Overwhelmed"
12. Disappointment
13. Doubt
14. Worry
15. Blame
16. Discouragement
17. Anger
18. Revenge
19. Hatred/Rage
20. Jealousy
21. Insecurity/Guilt/Unworthiness
22. Fear/Grief/Depression/Despair/Powerlessness

Your Body and its Connection to Mind, Spirit & Emotions

- Our cell tissue holds the energy patterns of one's attitudes and our belief systems.

- Positive and Negative experiences register a memory in cell tissue as well as in your energy field.

- Memory of experiences are stored in body tissue.

- Every thought continuously feeds every cell of your body.

- According to energy medicine, we are living history books. Our bodies contain our history.

- Day-to-Day Fearful or Bitter attitudes are biologically negative substances.

- All of our thoughts 1st enter our system as energy. This energy ends up in our body and cells.

- You can begin to cleanse your energy field by fasting and by a cleansing diet.

- Think of an Illness as a Power Disorder.

- We hold negative past emotions and experiences in our minds & bodies.

- Every thought that crosses our minds, every belief we nurture, every memory to which we cling translates into a positive or negative command to our bodies and spirits.

- If a person's spirit is impelled by Fear, then Fear returns to your energy field and to your body.

- What drains your spirit drains your body. What fuels your spirit fuels your body.

- Illness is the result of Imbalance.

- Be aware of the negative and lower frequency emotions such as fear, anger, judgment, envy, jealousy, resentment, hatred and impatience.

- Breathing creates awareness, space, and brings you into the Present moment. Create time to breathe. Create a few moments of inner stillness every day.

- Be Present. Be true to your inner purpose. Do not focus on the past or the future. Give the Present your full attention.

- Your Body and Energy System move naturally towards health.

The Power of Thought and the Law of Attraction

- Your every thought, every emotion, creates life.

- Everything you think now creates your moments to come, your future.

- All of your tomorrows are designed by your thoughts this very day.

- Listen to your feelings and intuitions. They are designed to help you.

- Thought is the ultimate creator. Whatever you think and then allow yourself to feel becomes the reality of your life.

- Accept that your life is constant growth and change, death and rebirth.

- What is the greatest way to manifest any desire? By speaking it forth from your spirit!

- Thought attracts, like a magnet, images you hold in your mind.

- Whatever you are thinking in your mind you tend to attract.

- Hold onto the thoughts you want. Thoughts become things!

- What you think about the most is what you will attract the most.

- Like attracts like. Make it clear in your mind what you want.

- If you affirm negative thoughts you will attract them. When you focus on negative attitudes, you will attract negativity.

- Do not focus on what you don't want. Most people think about what they don't want and it shows up. Focus on what you want.

- When you speak most of prosperity you will have it.

- When you speak most of success you will have it.

- You are the only one who creates your reality. Focus on what you want.

- A simple shift of emotions can change your day. Feel prosperous! Feel Happy!

- What you think and feel manifests. The more you feel good, the more you attract good.

- An affirmative thought is 100 times more powerful than a negative thought.

- Our feelings are our barometer. Whatever it is you are feeling is a perfect reflection of what is in the process of becoming. Bad vibes and negative emotions are telling you something.

- Positive emotions guide you towards alignment with the universe.

Steps towards Utilizing the Law of Attraction & Being Present

Step 1 - **Ask for what you want**. Doesn't have to be verbal. Visualize and affirm.

Step 2 - **The Answer & Believe** - the Universe will receive and answer your desire. You have to believe in what you ask, continue to focus and LET GO to the universe.

Step 3 - **Receive**. You must bring yourself into alignment with what you want.

Alignment = Joy, Passion, Enthusiasm towards what you want. The way you feel is everything.

Gratitude - Focus on what you have. Be thankful. This shifts your thinking.

Visualize - When you visualize, you materialize. Dwell on the end result. Feel the end result. Feel good about this result. It's the Feeling not just the visual thought that will attract your desire.

- When you have an inspired thought you have to act upon it.

- Success comes easily and frequently. Believe this about yourself.

- Stress causes Disease (Dis-ease) and Illness. Illness means there is something out of balance.

- People become what they think about.

- What you resist persists. Overweight?...focus on being healthy. Unhealthy?...focus on being healthy. Focus on what you want, not what you don't want.

- In order to attract success, you need to welcome it wherever it comes

- Let go of "the story"…the Past, and focus on the Present. This defines your future!

- Inner happiness is the Fuel for Success.

- Follow your Bliss. You are Source Energy. You are Divine!

- Align your outer purpose – with what you do with your inner purpose-awakening and staying awake. Your state of consciousness is the primary factor in what you do.

- The 3 energies of awakening and presence are acceptance, enjoyment and enthusiasm. One of these needs to be present whenever you are engaged in doing something.

- Take hold of your life. It belongs to you!

A Few Positive Concepts to Live By

1. Be in the Mystery of Life. Be open to each experience that you have.

2. The Origin of Suffering and Pain is Attachment to an outcome - past, present and future.

3. Law of Detachment - Happiness is letting go of any attachment or expectation.

4. We Create our own Reality. What you think manifests.

5. Visualize the Life you want. Feel the end result!

6. A Thought Alone can make change – Believe in yourself.

7. Simple Thoughts & Words can change things.

8. Our Thoughts affects our Reality.

9. Your Consciousness influences everyone around you.

10. Observe – Do not react with negative emotion.

11. Anger affects your consciousness & everyone around you.

12. Life is full of Possibilities...there is Magic before our eyes...there are no definite paths.

13. Unity – We Are One. We are all connected to the same universal energy source.

14. Take Time each day to Create Your Reality. Visualize and affirm this.

15. Practice Mindfulness. Be grateful of what you have today!

16. Ask yourself "What can I do to Serve others?" Giving brings you health & happiness.

17. Live in the Moment. Each event is a lesson.

18. You cannot avoid change. Embrace change as it makes you grow.

19. Avoid negative "low frequency" emotions such as anger, fear, jealousy and judgment.

20. Practice Forgiveness - Learn to let go of past wounds and move on to the Present.

21. Focus on the Present. Focus on Now.

22. Breathe. Practice deep breathing when stress & emotion overwhelm you.

Notes on Visualization, Affirmations, Meditation & Goals/Visions -

"Mental, Spiritual & Emotional Tune-Up" for your Success

It is essential that you take time 1-3 times per day or more to give yourself a "mental tune-up" and get the sub-conscious and the energy field working with you. For those of you who are not familiar with these techniques or who need a quick refresher here is some basic info to guide you. There are many great books and online articles on these subjects.

Affirmations - This is a positive thought, usually verbal, but it can also be in your mind. A good quote or a short sentence is best. It should always be positive and present. For example, "I am now healthy and fit" or "I am in shape, healthy, happy and fit " or " I am now ____ lbs (your ideal weight) and healthy". Repeat this as much as possible throughout the day. Feel it. Believe it…say it with emotion. Feel the joy and happiness. With the affirmation you can also include visualization.

Visualization - A guided inner vision of what you desire to become. See yourself healthy and fit. See yourself happy. Place yourself in a happy situation with your new look and healthy self. Use your affirmations as you visualize. Again feel it. Believe it. Feel the happiness. Feel the success. Continue this process at least 1-3 times per day, more if you want.

Meditation and Breathing - This is also important and can be part of your affirmations and visualization. It is important to be focused and calm. This is where breathing can help. Simple in and out breathing…take a breath in, let it go out, repeat. Focus on letting go and calming your mind and body. Do this and try to get other thoughts out of your mind. Focus just on the breathing. Take several minutes to be calm and relax, to let go, then start your affirmation and visualization with continued breathing. Do this as often as you can throughout the day with at least 2 special quiet times where you can focus. Meditation for 5-30 minutes is a great practice and I encourage it. Breathing and calm focus can also help you release stress…use it when you get tense or angry.

Create your Goals & Visions List - Along with these ideas and techniques you can become more organized and create a list of your goals and visions of who you want to be, or who you desire to become, or what you desire in your life. What you think about manifests. These goals need to be positive and in the present such as the examples in the affirmations' section. Make the list and write these down. Look at them often and start to incorporate them in your daily practice. Make them part of your affirmations and visualization. After a week or two you will begin to memorize them…they will slowly become part of your memory, which is connected to your sub-conscious and energy field.

Nature & Outdoors – Try to get fresh air and go for a hike or walk. Nature is a great way to relax and re-balance the system. Breathe and visualize while in the park or forest or by running water. Nature is inspirational and gives you positive healing energy.

Positive Affirmations with Food – Saying thanks and blessing our food is a very helpful technique. Saying "grace" or a prayer was at one time a common practice among many families. In these days many meals are eaten on the run or in front of the TV. Take time when you eat to be mindful and aware of eating. Start your meal with a positive affirmation towards the food. A simple "thank you for the food we are about to eat" works great. It is important to give thanks for two reasons. First, it makes you aware of the process of eating and the food itself. Second, it gets the positive intent and energy flowing to help you when you eat. It helps bring the Universe and the food to help with the process.

Note -I encourage you to look over these worksheets several times a week and incorporate the overall philosophies into your life and into your program. Pick your favorites and make your own list. This is part of your overall success and your transformation.

Section II –
The Natural Health &
Weight Loss Program

<u>Natural Health and Weight Loss Program</u>

<u>Introduction -</u>

Welcome to my program. Section I of my book gave you some important information to get your body, mind, spirit and emotions focused on overall health. Now you are ready and are about to begin a transforming journey. This program will help you succeed in losing the weight you desire, finding your optimum weight and gaining healthy body, mind, spirit and emotions. My program works. It is very straightforward and easy to follow, but please remember a key component is belief in yourself and in your success. I want to help you succeed, so continue to work focusing your thoughts and feelings towards your goals.

In this section I have included step-by-step easy to follow information for you to succeed, starting with my specific natural health and weight loss guidelines. In addition I have included a food chart and a resource guide at the end.

The info on the next several pages are important guidelines to my program. It is important that you follow these to the best of your ability. The more disciplined you are the better results you will have. If you need to "limit" some products instead of "avoid" them completely that is your choice, but be aware that my weight loss and health program will not be as effective. Please consult with me on what you would like to do. Keeping a diet journal and finding out which foods to avoid is the best strategy. Most of all, keep a positive attitude, believe in yourself and act upon that belief. You will see and feel the results.

My only medical recommendation is to have a qualified physician or health care professional monitor you if you have special conditions such as diabetes, high blood pressure, heart conditions, severe depression or another mental illness, are considered obese, or any other major health condition. I am not a trained doctor or certified nutritionist. I am an author, motivational speaker, counselor and life coach. I have extensive knowledge in health, nutrition and diet, but for special conditions that need to be monitored please seek the help of a qualified doctor or health care professional who supports the program. I would be more than happy to work with this professional to help you. This is an all natural program, it will change your body and your life, so I want you to be prepared.

And last, I want to again emphasize the importance of your belief and attitude. Our thoughts affect our reality. What you think and feel manifests. You have to think and feel positive. You have to believe in yourself and believe in your change. Positive affirmations and visualization of your success are essential for your transformation. This is a life changing program, but it is up to you. You are in charge! Think, feel and act with positive energy and you can do anything.

Please contact me if you need any assistance. I am here to help you succeed. To your health!

General Guidelines
Natural Health &
Weight Loss Program

✓ ***General Guidelines***

- Start each day with a positive affirmation and visualization of your success.

- Regular Organic herbal tea and filtered water are essential.

- Drink lots of Water. Filtered only.

- Drink Organic vegetable and natural juices for energy, fasting and hunger suppression.

- Organic and pure natural foods are essential.

- Eat natural or Organic lean proteins (chicken, fish, tofu, tempeh, beans and nuts are great).

- Eat fresh vegetables - green Organic vegetables and fresh salads are excellent.

- Eat more frequent smaller meals than the traditional large three meals a day. Try to eat or drink every 3-4 hours, but make it small. This keeps your energy going.

- Try to avoid Acidic foods as much as possible and keep your pH levels on the alkaline side. Your body needs Oxygen. Some good alkaline foods are fresh vegetables, fruits, beans and nuts. See the food list on page 92 for more information.

- Exercise 2 times daily - 30 min. minimum – important to sweat and increase heart rate. Work on muscle development also. Get Oxygen to your body regularly.

- Record daily in your personal journal your overall health, weight and energy levels.

- Avoid all processed and junk foods.

- Avoid or limit Dairy products.

- Avoid or limit Alcohol.

- Avoid or limit all Bread & Pasta products. Brown Rice or Spelt products are a possible substitute.

- Avoid or limit wheat, corn and potato products.

- Avoid or Limit Sugar products, especially processed refined sugar.

- Limit your caffeine intake. Limit and drink only Organic Coffee. Drink Organic herbal, black or green tea, or yerba mate as a substitute. Use only natural sweeteners and do not use dairy creamers.

- Do not eat too late in the evening. If possible exercise after your last big meal. If you are hungry in the evening drink tea, or a small protein, vegetable or fruit snack.

- Be aware of what foods make you "moody" and make you gain weight.

- Take a natural vitamin supplement. Preferably a liquid or powder so that you can digest it easily.

- Meditate, visualize, pray or take time each day to be quiet and focus.

- Ideally have a quiet time 2-3 times per day for at least 15 minutes.

- After optimal weight and health is reached re-introduce some of the avoidance foods into your diet, but very slowly and with the diet journal.

- Keep an accurate journal and awareness.

Natural Health Program – Weekly Guidelines

<u>Week 1 -</u>

1. <u>**Start with a Body Cleanse**</u> (7-14 day). Find a product at the natural foods store, there are many good ones. I will recommend three that I like - Total Body Rapid Cleanse by Renewlife (7 day), Whole Body Cleanse by Enzymatic Therapy (14 day) and 10 day Perfect Cleanse by Garden of Life. There are other good cleansers out there also, just make sure it is only 7-14 days and is natural. Follow this cleanse and drink lots of water and herbal tea. The 7 day works great for busy people, but follow it correctly. Some people may be sensitive to psyllium as a colon cleanser. There are alternatives to this type of cleanser. If you find you are constipated use a natural laxative tea for help to release your blockage. (see step 9) It is essential that you release as much toxins and build ups as possible to get your body working.

2. Attempt to curtail eating and fast as much as possible for several days during the cleanse. A Juice and Protein Fast is the best as it keeps your energy at a good level. Drink Organic Green, Vegetable & Fruit Juice.

3. If Fasting is difficult then eat 1-3 small meals a day to keep up your energy. Use the general guidelines as to what food to eat, but make it minimal for week 1 and the cleansing period. The less you can eat and the more you can fast the more toxins will be released from your system. Juices and liquids are better for the cleanse than solid food.

4. In general week 1 should be green vegetables and lean proteins only, along with some fruit and vegetable juice. Again, eating as little as possible is ideal so your body can cleanse and remove many of the toxins stored in there. Do not starve yourself though. Use tea and water as an appetite suppresser and cleanser. Drink green vegetable juice as a source of energy.

5. Small Protein meals such as raw almonds, tuna, salmon, skinless chicken, tofu and beans are all excellent, although limit solid food intake for week 1 & 2. Avoid eating too much fish and focus on Organic pure foods during your cleansing.

6. Avoid Wheat, Corn and Potatoes. Avoid Dairy Products and Alcohol. Use only Organic/natural low fat non dairy dressings with salads such as a vinaigrette dressing.

7. Drink lots of tea and water to help with appetite suppression and cleansing. Organic tea is best.

8. **<u>Exercise</u>** – Get lots of oxygen! Twice daily. At least 30 minutes of cardio and sweating in the AM and 30 minutes in the PM. AM workout can be the heavier one or vice versa. Be sure and raise heart rate and sweat! Put on an extra layer of clothing to help with sweating/cleansing. You do not have to go to the gym…you can run, walk, bike, swim, etc. Use this time also for visualizing health. Also do some weight lifting or muscle exercises. Lift simple free weights and focus on areas that your cardio exercise doesn't get to as much.

(arms and stomach for example) No weights? Lift some water jugs or something of weight. Do 3-4 sets of 30-60 reps 2-4 times per week. Get those muscles to work. This will help tone you and get your body working for you.

9. If constipated and blocked, which can occur with a cleanser, utilize a cleansing/flushing tea such as Yogi "Get Regular" or Traditional Medicinals "Smooth Move". Be cautious not to overuse these and follow directions. Get those toxins out of your body!

10. Keep an accurate health and diet journal.

11. Meditate, visualize, pray and take quiet time to be quiet and focus. This is very important for overall health and attitude. Your mind is the key to success.

12. Weigh before and after week 1 - you may not see a huge weight difference yet. Be patient and keep up the positive attitude.

Week 2 -

1. Continue Body Cleanse and Juice fast as directed. Utilize Juice fast during body cleanse.

2. Continue Steps 2-12 with the following notes and additions.

a. Juice fast is still important during week 2. Fast with juice in the morning and/or evening and supplement with 2-3 small protein-vegetable-fruit snacks during the day.

b. Drink plenty of water and tea for appetite suppression and cleansing. There are many good Organic teas that are very helpful for this purpose. My favorites are from Yogi Tea and Traditional Medicinals.

c. Eat as necessary small snacks to keep up your energy. Keep in mind that you are cleansing your system so do not overload it with solid food.

d. For snack foods eat Organic baby carrots, celery, apples, raw almonds, sunflower seeds, cooked tofu, etc. Make sure and eat light snacks more often than large portions and remember that most of these products contain natural sugars so limit your intake.

e. Continue to avoid all the foods mentioned in the Guidelines, the Food list starting on page 89 and Week 1 steps. Be very careful not to re-introduce the "avoidance" foods. The more you can keep these products out of your diet, the better results of weight loss and health. After week 4 we will begin to re-introduce a few selective foods to see if your body will assimilate them in a healthy way.

f. Utilize cleansing/constipation tea if necessary, but do not overuse or use daily.

g. Monitor your weight, energy levels and overall progress. Use your diet journal.

h. Continue positive spiritual or psychological practice.

Week 3-4

1. Continue Steps 2 - a. through h. from Week 2 guidelines.

2. If you desire increase meal size by adding more lean natural proteins, green vegetables and salads, healthy snack foods as mentioned on page 85, and fruit juice.

3. Monitor any food or juice increase carefully. Use diet journal and be aware of any changes.

Week 5-16

1. Continue Steps 1-3 of week 3-4.

2. This is the time, if you are losing weight and progressing, to possibly re-introduce a few select products into your diet. This is my recommendation -

a. <u>Organic brown rice</u> is the best carbohydrate to re-introduce into your meals. Start with this product and monitor your overall progress. Do not overuse…minimize use of any carbohydrate.

b. Be very careful re-introducing any of the other avoidance foods into your diet. Try one type of food at a time and in small portions. Try this for a week having it in your diet. Try it in 1-3 meals in a week and monitor. If you are still making positive progress than most likely this food will be okay, but do not increase portions quickly and use sparingly until you are certain it is part of your overall plan.

c. In general I would continue to minimally use or avoid altogether the following - dairy products, wheat products, breads and flours, pasta, alcohol, refined sugars, any processed or refined foods, and any preservative or artificial additives. Natural corn and potatoes can be re-introduced into your system slowly, noting any energy changes and weight gain, although use these foods sparingly if possible. Fresh organic corn and organic red potatoes are best. Spelt or rice flour products are also a possibility if you want to eat flour type products. Again get used to using these products sparingly if possible. If possible avoid regular wheat products or use sparingly.

d. This is an essential time to be patient and go very slow with re-introducing foods into your diet. It is essential that you keep your diet journal current and make notes on any changes.

e. It is also essential that you keep up your spiritual or psychological practice by making it part of your day. Visualizing, meditating, praying, affirmations…these are all important health tools and should be continued regularly.

Beyond - Maintaining your Health and Weight

Once you have reached your goal you will be able to experiment with certain foods to see if they are good for you or not. This is where your journal comes in handy. Be aware of what foods affect your energy levels, your overall weight, as well as your attitude. You can eat certain foods on special occasions and still keep your health. Reintroducing unhealthy and processed foods into your diet on a regular basis is not recommended.

Use the General Guidelines from page 79 and continue to eat healthy. <u>**A few reminders**</u> -

- Continue to drink lots of filtered water, tea and natural juices. Your body is mostly made of water and you need to replenish and cleanse the system often.

- Try to cleanse and juice fast 2-4 times a year if possible…a minimum of once a year is highly recommended

- Avoid Processed, refined & junk foods as much as possible.

- Avoid Preservatives and artificial flavors and colors in food and drink.

- Avoid saturated fatty oils and foods.

- Eat Organic and Natural Food & Liquids.

- Eat lots of Fresh Organic Vegetables, Fruits and Lean Proteins.

- Exercise daily. Keep that blood and heart flowing. Keep the oxygen levels up. Work on your muscle development also.

- Continue your spiritual or psychological practice of visualization, prayer or meditation.

- Breathe - take time to release your stress and practice breathing.

Organic & Natural Foods – Why this is Essential to your Health!

Toxins and chemicals in our bodies is one of the biggest factors in health and weight loss. I can't emphasize this enough. Processed foods with chemicals are simply not good for you. If you are going to lose permanent weight and have good health you need to limit or avoid chemicals in your food. These chemicals affect us in many ways. A pure natural diet is the best thing you can do for yourself. The easiest way to do this is to buy and eat only Organic foods. As a second best and when 100% Organic is not feasible eat all natural. It is very easy to look at product labels. And it is not difficult to find out what is all natural and Organic and what is not. Be your best advocate for health. There are thousands of great Organic and natural products out there. You have great choices. Even when you are in a mainstream grocery store you have healthy choices. Fresh vegetables and fruits are obviously the best choice. All natural lean proteins are also a key. Try and look for Organic products as much as possible. Yes, Organic food cost more, but what is the total cost of your health over years to come? And why are people so overweight? I hope you have made the connection between health and what you eat. You cannot eat high fat and high sugar foods laced with additives and chemicals. You are what you put in your body. Work hard towards eating Organic and all natural…this will help your body, mind, spirit and emotions in amazing ways.

Food List - General Guidelines

Note - It is very important that you find out what foods work for you and which do not. Keep an accurate diet journal. Everyone's blood type, metabolism and energy systems are unique. The list below is a general guideline of what foods work the best and what foods you should avoid or eat sparingly. Experiment with certain foods and see if they give you health or not.

<u>**Foods -**</u>

<u>**Water**</u> – Drink lots of water. Flush that system out regularly and replenish your body fluids. Drink only filtered or spring water. Avoid unfiltered city water as much as possible as it contains many chemicals and heavy metals. Buy a quality water filter. Water is one of the best things you can do for your body. Do not forget to drink several glasses a day. Juice and tea are a great addition as they are mostly water.

<u>**Proteins**</u> - Fish, Organic Tofu, Natural Chemical-Free Skinless Chicken, Organic Eggs, Organic Nuts (almonds, sunflowers), Beans and Legumes. Lean Organic beef and other meats are okay when used sparingly, but lean meats are the best. Fish is great, but do not eat it every day as there are many trace chemicals and heavy metals in ocean fish. Wild caught Salmon is a great source of protein though and has healthy oils. A Natural Protein powder can also be used as a supplement for your need for protein, but limit use of this and make certain it is all natural.

Vegetables - Green vegetables are best - kale, broccoli, greens, etc. Every fresh vegetable is good for you. Organic is the best. Carrots and Celery are great snack foods. Eat lots of fresh vegetables. Lightly steamed is okay. Organic onions, tomatoes & peppers are also a great way to flavor food.

Fruits - Organic fruits are great for you. They do contain sugar though, so use them for snacks and quick energy, not for an entire meal.

Dressings and Condiments - Avoid creamy milk based dressings. Use vinaigrettes and low fat dressings. Make sure they are natural with no preservatives. Newman's and Annie's dressings have some great choices. Avoid mayonnaise. Non dairy Veganaise is better. Organic mustard, ketchup, salsa and chutney are great low fat additions to foods.

Natural Carbohydrates - Organic Brown Rice is the best carbohydrate. Avoid wheat, corn and potatoes as much as possible or use sparingly, in particular wheat. Spelt is much better, but still has gluten. Organic red potatoes can be eaten sparingly as can fresh corn. Avoid breads, flour and pasta products as much as you can, in particular refined products.

Breads. Pasta and Flour Products - Rice Pasta or Spelt are the best, rice being the preferred choice. Whole grain breads and flour products are okay, but use sparingly. Whole wheat or Spelt tortillas only, but use sparingly. Natural Rice wraps (used for eggs rolls) are also a good substitute if you need a wrap or tortilla. In general avoid breads and pasta or eat smaller portions and/or use sparingly.

Eggs and Dairy - As a general rule use dairy sparingly or avoid if possible. Organic eggs can be a good source of protein. Low fat cheese can also be used to flavor food, although use sparingly. Avoid fatty dairy products such as sour cream, half-n-half, whole milk or regular processed cheese. Try to buy Organic and natural products. Use soy or almond cheese and soy creamer as a substitute.

Alcohol - Limit or avoid alcohol as much as possible. Alcohol has lots of sugar and also makes you eat more. Physically and psychologically it is additive and not very healthy. If you drink, limit your intake and do not drink every day. Give your body a few days off to cleanse. Organic wine and beer are the first choice. Avoid mixed drinks with high sugar and cream.

Sugar - White processed sugar and corn syrup are not recommended. Avoid soda. If you have to use sugar in something, natural Organic cane sugar is the best. Use agave sweetener (available at natural food stores) or honey. Do not use chemical sweeteners of any kind.

Juice & Tea - Organic Natural Juice and Tea are essential for your health. Herbal and Green Tea are a great cleanser and appetite suppressor. Green Juice with spirilina, algae, green vegetables, wheat grass, etc are great for you. Carrot and beet juice are also good, and any combination of vegetables and fruits. Try to avoid high sugar smoothies, instead find a fruit vegetable mix. Buy a juicer and juice your own Organic juices. Organic or Natural Fruit juice is also good, but do not overuse as it contains high amounts of sugar. Avoid carbonated soda as much as possible.

Caffeine - Limit your caffeine intake. Caffeine causes stress and raises your heart rate. It also can be an energy drain if you are addicted to it. Coffee is highly acidic. Organic coffee is okay, but limit consumption and avoid processed sugars and dairy creamers. Substitute herbal, black and green tea or yerba mate. Drink lots of Organic herbal tea. There are some great flavorful Organic teas to choose from.

Soy Products - Organic soy is a great product for most people. It is a great source of protein and a great substitute for most dairy and meat products. Some people's metabolisms are different with soy though, so monitor this with your journal and use sparingly if you feel it is not benefiting your weight loss or energy levels. Otherwise eat lots of Organic soy products. It is a great meat substitute. Look online for how to prepare and cook soy. For those sensitive to soy try tempeh and/or miso as it can be easier to digest.

Processed and Refined Foods - Avoid junk food of any kind. This food is full of saturated fat, refined sugars and carbohydrates, and chemicals.

Spices - Avoid any refined spices. Use Organic and natural spices only. Spices such as garlic, pepper, onion, ginger, rosemary, dill, paprika, cayenne, thyme, oregano, marjoram, curry, etc and a variety of Eastern and Indian mixes are a great low fat/low salt way to flavor food. Natural salt is okay, but use sparingly.

Cooking and Oils, etc - Use Organic natural oils only. Do not use butter for cooking. You can utilize Organic Ghee (a clarified butter) if you need the butter flavor. Use appropriate oils for high temperature. Olive, sunflower, safflower, canola, grape seed, these are all good oils. There are many lists online that give you the benefits of each oil. Use all oils sparingly. If possible do not fry food.

Vitamins – Vitamin supplements are an excellent idea. I would recommend a liquid or powder supplement during this diet as it is easier to digest and assimilate into your system. You can get most of your vitamins from good food, but I am a firm believer in supplements. Make sure you only use an all natural or Organic vitamin supplement. There are many great products out there, but ask a nutritionist for the best all natural product.

Acidic vs Akaline Food & Drink –
Excess Acidic foods in general are toxic to the body. Although they can be eaten in smaller quantities the body likes more foods and the pH of your body on the alkaline side. This is a guideline, not a rule. Coffee, red meat, sausage, alcohol, any sugar product, ketchup, any white processed carbohydrate, soft drinks and most canned food are examples of Acid-forming foods and

drink. Alkaline–forming products include most vegetables, fruits, almonds, sunflower seeds, garlic, beans and most edible grasses and their juices. Most of us eat in such a way that our bodies are highly acidic. This depletes oxygen in our bodies and can cause illness and disease. If we can keep our pH levels at around 7.4 we are considered healthy. Natural clean water is around 7 pH, which is neutral. Acid is 1pH, Alkaline is 14pH. Coffee is highly acidic so it is best to limit your intake. Regular exercise and stress reduction also helps with acid reduction in the body. Overall if you follow my guidelines and program you will be avoiding or limiting most acidic-forming foods.

Restaurant Foods - Most restaurants serve food that is high sugar, fatty, non-Organic or not natural, and is full of preservatives. However, there are many progressive restaurants that are changing this. Be aware when you eat out what you are eating. Try to avoid any foods that contain preservatives and chemicals. Avoid fried foods of any kind. Go light on breads and carbohydrates. Eat light when you go out. Limit your portions. Be aware that you are probably eating foods that will bring toxins, processed sugars and fats into your body.

Conclusion – *This list is not exclusive and gives you general guidelines to follow*. I did not list every type of food, but it should give you a good idea as to what is generally healthy and what is not. Again, you need to see what works for you. Experiment and keep up your diet journal. Read and look online for more information on foods and their connection to health. To your health!

Natural Health & Weight Loss Sample Chart

<u>**On Page 99 is a 7 day sample chart for you to develop on your own.**</u> **The page is somewhat small to make a great chart, but feel free to copy the concept. You can make a table by hand or with the computer and monitor your daily progress.**

<u>*Also it is very important to keep an Attitude & Diet Journal for additional comments and notes*</u>

Do not be afraid to write down your thoughts & feelings. This is your journal and chart. It also helps you keep organized and monitor your goals.

Natural Health & Weight Loss Sample Chart

Date	Weight	Attitude-Energy	Notes

RESOURCES & WEBSITES

Resources & Websites

The people and websites listed on the next page are a few teachers, books and DVDs that have been inspirational to my work and to my success, in particular the body, mind, spirit and emotional connection.

Check out their websites and their various books and DVDs. <u>This is by no means a complete list of people who are leaders in this area</u>, but these people below are part of a very strong movement of healers, counselors, philosophers, scientists and business people that are conscious and aware of a movement in which Eckhart Tolle refers to as "The New Earth".

I encourage you to explore and read additional material from these authors and from others in this field. Take time to read as much material as you can. There is so much good information out there.

Feel free to contact me personally with your questions and comments. Let me know how you are doing.

To your Health and your Success!

Brian M Heater
bheater@transformingourselves.com

Resources & Websites

Author , Book or DVD	Website Address
The Secret	http://thesecret.tv/
Dr Joe Vitale	http://www.mrfire.com/
Deepak Chopra	http://www.chopra.com/
Eckhart Tolle	http://www.eckharttolle.com/
Esther & Jerry Hicks	http://www.abraham-hicks.com
Ramtha	http://ramtha.com
Caroline Myss	http://myss.com
Thich Nhat Hanh	http://www.parallax.org & http://www.iamhome.org
Barbara Brennan	http://barbarabrennan.com/
What the Bleep Do We Know!?	http://www.whatthebleep.com/
James A Ray	http://jamesray.com/
Neale Donald Walsch	http://nealedonaldwalsch.com/
A Course In Miracles	http://www.acim.org/
Alternative Health Info	http://totalhealthbreakthroughs.com/
Dr Wayne Dyer	http://www.drwaynedyer.com/
James Twyman	http://www.emissaryoflight.com
Dalai Lama	http://www.dalailama.com/
Andrew Weil, MD	http://www.drweil.com/
You – The Owners Manual	http://youtheownersmanual.com

For more Information on our Books, Programs, Events & Blog

www.StarttheRevolutionWithin.com

www.RevolutionStartsWithin.com

www.Transformingourselves.com

www.ingramcontent.com/pod-product-compliance
Lightning Source LLC
Chambersburg PA
CBHW060635290526
45793CB00001B/253